PANDORA'S BOX
THE DRAMA OF SCHIZOPHRENIA

INTRODUCTION

We are all part of life's wa ⁞ are unaware of how very damag uate diagnosis of the human condition in general and of illness in particular. I suffer from schizophrenia and when I tried to reach out for assistance in order to recover, I found none was available other than drug therapy.

I recognised the seriousness of my illness and despite the wall of silence I met with from the medical establishment, I set about my own therapy to get to the roots of my condition.

In this book, I relate my experiences of schizophrenia together with a commentary. This is an honest confrontation with my unconscious. Knowledge and acknowledgement of illness has been the process that has enabled me to cope with this devastating and socially unattractive illness. I hope others who may read this book will gain some insight into the perplexing world of schizophrenia.

PANDORA'S BOX

Pandora was very lovely but very inquisitive. She longed to know what was in the mysterious box she had been forbidden to open. One day she could not resist peeping inside. Out of the box flew all the evils that plague the world – disease, old age, war and death. As Pandora stared in horror at the empty box, one last thing emerged. It was Hope and it meant that the world should never despair.

Pandora's box is a good analogy to make with my mind. During my experiences of schizophrenia, all kinds of terrors have emerged from my mind but I have never given into despair because I always had hope and refused to believe I was mad.

It is now well established medically that schizophrenia is a disease related to abnormalities in the structure and function of the human brain. How can I describe schizophrenia? Imagine you have awakened from a frightening nightmare:

PANDORA'S BOX

* * * * *

THE DRAMA OF SCHIZOPHRENIA

A personal experience of schizophrenia

by

Carole Buckingham

For my family and friends – past and present

I shut my eyes in order to see

Paul Gaugin

PREFACE

Dear Reader,

I wrote this narrative in 2003 and we are now many years hence. As I enter old age and the years creep by, it is tempting to think that my life's work is done. However, I still remember the times when I was at my weakest and most vulnerable. I would like to share my insights of those times with you. In 2003, I was unable to find a publisher for my book but thanks to the advances of modern technology it is possible today to self-publish a book without too much hassle. I believe that what I have written is still as relevant as it was 16 years ago. Good reader, please step into the mind of a schizophrenic. I did not surrender to my illness and what I have to say matters and sheds light on a deeply misunderstood illness.

Carole

October 2019

relief, it was just a dream. But what if you were not asleep and you are fully conscious and that nightmare is your reality. You hear voices. They taunt you. You fear for yourself and perhaps all humanity. You see things that are not there. You are bombarded with thoughts and you believe you have no privacy of mind. Your senses become more acute and the sound of a car or the babble of voices is intolerable. People misunderstand you. They cannot reach you because they do not understand the road that you are travelling. Yes, it is a nightmare and there is no release with the morning.

There is as yet no cure for schizophrenia. It is a way of life. A gradual process of recovery and rehabilitation often marked by setbacks. Recovery is not getting rid of the symptoms but being able to face what has happened to you.

Like Pandora, I was inquisitive. I felt a need to make sense of the experience. Actually, schizophrenia did not drive me insane; it drove me to delve deeper into my mind. The multitudes of thoughts that bombard my mind during an attack go from the very personal to my fears for all humanity. In many ways my illness has given me a philosophical insight into life that I would not otherwise have made. My change in perception has led me to a greater freedom of mind and imagination.

Voices and images that arise in the unconscious world of our dreams are considered natural and normal. If they cross over into our conscious world they are viewed with fear and the person labelled 'deranged'. Often there is no analysis into the contents of psychosis for fear of giving credence to delusions or provoking another attack. I think analysis would lead to finding common grounds between patients. A schizophrenic's behaviour is more intelligible that what most of the medical establishment would suppose. Unless you can confront your unconscious world you cannot understand the true nature of your condition and the drugs you are prescribed will only suppress your symptoms.

I try to analyse the surreal world of my psychoses and I hope with discernment. This has given me a greater awareness of myself and the world in which we live. I may in many respects be a slave to my condition but my attitude towards my illness has changed. This has enabled me to grow and move forward.

The psyche is a complex structure of which the conscious mind is one aspect. Beneath the conscious mind are the manifold levels of what is termed the unconscious. The conscious mind influences the unconscious mind and the unconscious mind influences the conscious mind. The unconscious can be a wellspring of creative material and inspiration. However, it also contains material that can be very disturbing. There are destructive forces which can shatter our sense of who we are, our familiar habits of behaviour, our sense of morality and rationality.

What happens during a schizophrenic crack-up is that we are plunged into the world of our unconscious – an inner world and the experience can be for better and for worse. It can be a terrible period of mental upheaval from which not everyone will emerge.

* * * * *

EPISODE 1

PARIS SUMMER 1984

MY FIRST EPISODE OF SCHIZOPHRENIA

I woke up early one morning to experience a pain ripping though my brain. I started to hear angelic voices in my head. I had suddenly become telepathic. I had recently broken up with my American boyfriend. The voices told me to forget him. I was going to meet somebody special – a prince. I got dressed and followed the directions the voices gave me. I wandered in the streets looking for my prince. I eventually ended up outside a church at Porte St Cloud. The voices told me to enter. I angrily refused. I felt they had been playing games with me. I told them I was not going in the church. I was a non-practising Catholic at that time and had left the church because Roman Catholicism had been the cause of war, intolerance and corruption. I connected the Inquisition with the Holocaust. I stamped my foot and walked away. I had gone someway down the road when suddenly I heard the church bell ring for mass. A tremendous force, which I can only describe as a hurricane, scooped me up and threw me back to the church. "You will go in" was the message I heard. I was pretty awe struck. I felt I had met God the Almighty. I didn't know where the entrance to the church was so I followed an old lady limping with a stick. I listened to the mass in silence. So, this was the prince I had been taken to meet – Jesus Christ.

I walked home in a confused state. When I reached my flat, I hunted out my copy of the New Testament and opened it. I randomly picked a page and the piece of scripture staring me in the face was:

"Why do you look at the speck in your brother's eye and take no notice of the log in your own... You hypocrite...'

This piece of scripture was very appropriate as I was very good at criticising others but never thought of my own failings. Shortly after that I descended into a dark hell to do battle with demons. I saw images of evil and felt satanic influences were at war with my mind. I was not fighting a human enemy.

I changed from my pink dress into grey – the colour of repentance. Next morning, I again went to mass in my grey attire – grey slacks and grey duffle coat underneath I had only my underwear. The girl in the pew in front was blond and wore a pink dress. I was a brunette in grey. We shook hands at the sign of peace. I felt she was my opposite. She was taking the high road; I was taking the low road. I couldn't partake in communion as I was in a state of mortal sin through having missed mass for several years.

After mass, I went to a nearby bench. A gang of Italian gangsters appeared across the road from me. They were led by my ex husband's uncle who was allegedly in the Mafia. He had come to kill me for deserting my husband. I stood up in the face of his gun and confronted by my courage he lowered the weapon.

I was woken from this reverie by a small unpleasant man in a car who asked me to go for a ride with him. What he saw in me I do not know. I looked a wreck in my sackcloth and ashes and I was shocked this should happen by a church.

"Je ne suis pas une prostituée", I told him - I am not a prostitute.

My voices became capricious. Back at the flat, I was ordered in a colour code sequences to get rid of all my belongings - clothes, jewellery, furniture etc. I broke my sofa bed to physically symbolise my rupture with my boyfriend. The concierge helped me dispose of the furniture. I threw out all but three books (an autograph book with goodwill messages; my copy of the New Testament and a black and gold bound copy of the complete works of Shakespeare which I had never taken the time to dip into). I had given in to Mammon – that is to say modern civilisation. I was a materialist girl in a materialist world and by this radical renunciation of worldly goods, I was getting back to true values. The voices said I needed to learn discipline, so every time I disobeyed them, I was punished by electric shocks to my brain.

In a brief moment of lucidity, I left the flat remembering what the nuns had told us on our last day of school: "If you are ever in trouble go and see a priest". The church was 5 minutes from my flat and I begged for help. The priest told me to go to a hospital but on entering the hospital I was too frightened to stay. I didn't think my problem was medical. I went to see another priest his answer was: "Come back for catechism lessons in a fortnight.". I wandered around Paris hallucinating. I saw terrifying images of evil. Only music gave me any comfort and I sang hymns at the top of my voice in an attempt to jam the hostile transmissions. I asked for sanctuary at three convents – I was given the 'miraculous medal' (a catholic token of piety which promises help to those who wear it) and was told that Mary would watch over me.

Eventually on the third day of my disturbed state, I found myself a little before midnight in front of the Café Étoile, a stone's though away from the Place Charles de Gaulle and the Arc de Triomphe. The voices had won. They called me "dumbbell". I did not see the connection. But then they said: "runt" and I did understand that word. An immense force pushed me forward towards the Tomb of the Unknown Warrior beneath the Arc de Triomphe. I started on my way for I feared further bouts of 'electric shock' treatment. As I neared the massive roundabout that rings the arch and tomb, a dawning came to me; I was being used as a pawn by the 'Powers That Be' to decide the future fate of the world. It was a game they played every now and then. If I allowed them to lead me to the tomb there would be an apocalyptical world war. (I know this is all sheer paranoia but at the time it was frightening and very real). Back in 1984, the Soviet Union was seen as the grizzly threat but the message I received was that due to serious economic recession, starvation would hit Africa and spread to China. The outcome would be war and the consequences unspeakable. I wrestled with the force – I must not reach the tomb. I believed the fate of the entire world depended on me. On mass there is much to dislike about the human race; but faced with the prospect of its annihilation, I wanted to save it. Above all, I did not want those I loved to suffer.

I discovered I still had a will and despite this force majeure, drew back from the brink. When midnight passed, the compelling force relented and I was told I was the last but one. The last but one what? I only knew I was the last but one because I was standing at the second road from the Tomb of the Unknown Warrior. THEY would put us with us a little longer – 'Apocalypse Now' had been postponed.

I went and sheltered under some scaffolding down a side road opposite what appeared to me as a magnificent mansion. A voice from within this palace spoke to me. I was told there would emerge a future leader. The voice posed a question: if the choice was mine, from which rung on the social ladder should HE come. I said the lowest – the poor working class as I was hoping for a re-run of the Jesus story but this time with a happy ending for this world. The voice derided me: the ranks of the rich and powerful make the world go around – HE must come from amongst them. "No", I cried from beneath the scaffolding: "A future Saviour should be born in a stable"; meaning today's equivalent. I was given to understand that my naïve fixed beliefs were rendering me a lame brain and this blight was illustrated graphically by the green man on the traffic lights starting to limp. I needed educating. I pleaded with the voice: "Why is this happening to me? Why!". The reply was phrased in a question: Was there any other way?". I was left standing humiliated under the scaffolding. I felt the voices had been laughing at my innocence.

The next morning, I tried to find my way to the British Embassy but the whole city was whirling by me and I could not find it. I wended my way back to the church and demanded that a priest confess me as I felt near to death. I then wandered towards Passy and the office where I was found by Danielle, a Swiss colleague who was kind enough to get me to hospital.

* * * * *

My French doctor prescribed a cocktail of drugs to treat my condition. At this point I was unaware it was schizophrenia. The drugs were very disabling. I felt like one of the walking dead. My life was one of paralysis and stagnation. Six months later I left Paris to be cared for by my family in London, but before leaving France, and on my own initiative I stopped taking the drugs and experienced an immediate recovery. I enjoyed a normal life again. It is no use treating the mind if the side effects disable the body. However, in time I was to relapse.

* * * * *

COMMENTARY 1

The foregoing is a description of my first experience of schizophrenia when I was living and working in Paris back in 1984. Psychotic fantasies are very similar to dreams. I maintain that the fund of images that confuse my mind during a psychotic attack are not senseless neurotic obsessions but in fact have meaning. The guilt feelings I had about my failed marriage are acted out in the early part of my account by my encounter with my husband's 'Mafia' uncle. I saw divorce as a stigma – a sin against social and religious convention. There is my desire to stop a Third World War. At the time of my illness the arms race was in full flow and Armageddon could have been around the corner. So, psychosis can have a relation to observable reality as well as being an expression of imagination. I was trying to serve humanity and at the same time this gave my own life dignity, meaning and purpose. In reality, I was an insignificant individual, maladapted and helpless in a reckless modern-day world.

What is normal? What is mad? They are relative terms. After all millions of normal Christians believe in the actual fact of the Virgin Birth and this is a concept that could not possibly be true in any scientific sense. Yet not all Christians are mad! I maintain that if an idea is psychologically true; it can be considered a true concept.

It is evident from my account of psychosis that my Roman Catholic upbringing has left an indelible mark on my mind. The voices challenged my naive understanding of religion. This set me on a quest for truth and I now see Christ's mystical birth and resurrection as mythological and esoteric rather than fact. However, I do believe there is a power in the universe to whom I shall return.

My first experience of schizophrenia was a perilous journey into darkness. I saw evil as a reality and who after the death camps of Nazi Germany can deny evil is a reality. I am sure many of the solid citizens of Germany never thought they were participating in evil, but nonetheless they were instruments of evil. In truth we all participate in evil only the degree is different. On the whole it is not human nature that is evil, but we are made evil by circumstances.

Today it is easier to think that evil does not exist or that it is a temporary aberration. This excuses us of moral obligation. The fact is when I was ill, I saw terrifying images of evil and still today because of my sensitivity, I censor what I watch on film and television. Evil is popular at the movies but evil like good is a reality that works through men and women in our ordinary everyday world. Why do I mention evil, because psychosis like a film, is a series of sounds and images that tell a story. Psychosis can be a horror story and in the inner recesses of the human mind there are destructive forces of which we are not consciously aware. During a schizophrenic crack-up you can easily be swamped by them, as indeed I was. I mention them because you cannot defeat or better transfigure these hidden forces unless you are aware of them. You have to accept what has happened to you and not be dominated by the encounter. How else can you find healing? I believe it is possible to interpret the experience with reason which leads to a greater self-knowledge and can only strengthen you should further relapses occur. There is a need to make sense of the experience.

* * * * *

EPISODE 2

LONDON AUTUMN 1985

It was the blessing. The end of Mass. The sending forth back into the world. Since my episode of psychosis in Paris, I had returned to the Church and took my religious observation earnestly. I conformed to all the rules and even beyond. Not out of love of God but out of fear of him. In Paris I had met God and the Devil and been vanquished by both. But my fearful service was not what He wanted. At least that was what I was given to understand.

"Have you learned nothing from your previous experience?" the voice said. It was God talking to me. True I had tried to blank out my previous psychotic experiences.

I ran out of the church, past my father waiting to take mum and me home and raced down the road. Mum and dad followed in the car. They must not catch me. Mum was a witch and dad Rumpelstiltskin. Seeing my parents as characters out of folklore frightened me. I knocked on a door to plead for help. No-one answered. Mum and Dad got out of the car. I could not outrun a motor machine. I pushed violently passed them.

I ran back up to the Church. The power of religion was my only hope. The Parish Priest saw me in the Presbytery.

"I'm possessed. Something evil is overpowering me. I want to be exorcised."

I felt I was Beelzebub – the devil. I was fighting for possession of my body. The priest gave me the sacrament for the sick and I grew calmer. He offered me a lift home but I refused. I needed air and space.

Outside, I took off my camel coat and left it on a wall. I was lighter now. Neasden became the deserts of Arabia. Within it was hidden a mystical jewel - Me. I ran home in a state of ecstasy. The wind blew in my hair and my eyes were raised loft ward to the sky.

Only mum was at home. Dad had gone to the police with a photograph of me in order to seek their assistance. I needed to rest and went upstairs. Disorderly thoughts were racing round my head and would give me no rest. I stayed in my room.

The next day because I had not come out of my delirium mum called the doctor. I was in terrible anguish. There were a multitude of bats in my belfry. Time stood still. I was in a time warp. There was no past and no future – just an eternity of now. This was hell. Normally the present moment passes us by without we take the least bit of notice. But I was in a non-stop now. I restlessly paced up and down the stairs as a means of dissipating the energies that were bubbling up inside me.

The doctor came and went. He left a green pill. I would never swallow it. It was poison.

Father Casey who was also my Godfather came down to visit me.

"Yin Yang Yung or Mao Tse Tung". Much to his annoyance I kept repeating the words. This message had come into my head during a recent dizzy spell in W H Smiths the booksellers. The 'Yung' had led me phonetically to 'Jung' the Swiss author and psychologist. I had bought a pile of his books but had not yet read a word of his writings.

During my delirium, I had written automatically the word 'Ariel' which I translated to aerial. I was an aerial for the Gods and my message was for the Pope.

"Yin, Yang, Yung or Mao Tse Tung".

This was an esoteric way of saying that unless the world finds balance there will be war with communist China.

The message went on:

"Lot says: "You may keep my daughters but leave my sons alone!"

I was a son of the biblical Lot. This my mind interpreted to mean that as a son of Lot, I was not to be muzzled by the Church.

"The Pope has the keys"

was the final part of the message.

The keys of St Peter are an insignia of the Pope.

After I had given the first part of the message to Father Casey who of course thought I was talking gibberish, he proceeded to speak to me of how it was impossible to understand suffering and how the British prisoners of War had suffered many ordeals at the hands of the Japanese. It was obvious that Father Casey did not know how to relate to me. My mind was on the message and the possibilities of another war.

That night I had the hallucination that I was the sleeping Arthur of Britain floating peacefully on a barge on a celestial river with St Gabriel, St Michael and St Raphael watching over me. I was a sleeper to be awaken when needed. An aerial to transmit a warning but I did not know who the receptor would be. I was a link in a chain.

* * * * *

A doctor experienced in mental health came to see me and advised that I should be sent to Shenley, the nearest mental hospital. Shenley was a vast cluster of buildings set in lovely surroundings. Rather like a small village. I adored wandering round the expanse of grass and trees. There was a tea bar and a library. I was in a large room with about six other women. We quickly struck up a friendship.

One Sunday, we attended morning service at the Anglican chapel. Although I was brought up Roman Catholic, my father was an Anglican and I had attended Anglican services before. The chapel was large and my friends and I sat at the back. At the front I saw Nanny, my dead Grandmother, she was kneeling as if in prayer. Everyone sang and spoke at a sluggish rate. It was as if a record was playing at the wrong speed.

On the whole, I enjoyed the rest at Shenley. My doctor was a lovely warm woman who I liked instantly. I told her I had been ill before in Paris and she said she would write to the American Hospital in Paris for my notes. The doctor prescribed stelazine. This time I did not have the disabling side-effects I experienced in Paris. However, stelazine is a heavy-duty drug which can have serious side-effects if taken over long periods of time but at least I found I could function normally.

Gradually, I stabilized and was sent home. It was then that depression set in. At the hospital, I took each day as it came and gave no thought to the future. I now realised that my condition was a recurring one and I would have to face up to the reality of my illness and not try and blank it out as I did in Paris.

When I saw my doctor in outpatients, I was still rather low. They had received no response from the American Hospital in Paris and she suggested I write which I did to no avail. She also referred me for psychotherapy. This took a few months to come through.

In the meantime, I read Carl Gustav Jung's autobiography from which I learned there was such a thing as the unconscious mind which prompted me to go around the bookshops in London seeking books on mental health. My reading led me to the conclusion that I was suffering from a condition called schizophrenia.

My doctor at outpatients changed. I now saw an Asian woman doctor and I asked her if I was suffering from schizophrenia. She confirmed my diagnosis but said that mine was not one of the worst forms. I asked anxiously if she could give me information on my condition and how best to cope with it. She replied: "We still don't know how the brain works."

I had come to a dead end.

I asked to see the Consultant. I needed help and advice on how to deal with my condition.

He said: "What can I do for you?"

I replied: "I was hoping you could tell me what could be done."

The Consultant got impatient and said if I did not know what I wanted there was nothing he could do. I felt rather confused and embarrassed in his presence. I was hoping for help and reassurance. I got what amounted to a flea in my ear.

Psychotherapy was my last hope. Perhaps I might be able to join a group and learn of other people's experiences. The day of the appointment came and I arrived at the clinic in good time. But they were not expecting me. It appeared they had not received my confirmation of attendance or the duly filled in questionnaire that I had sent.

"Are you telling me the Post Office don't do their job properly", the doctor lanced at me. My experience was that the Post Office did an efficient job. I had never lost any letters and I told him so. We had got off to a bad start.

I found the doctor aggressive and when he asked me if I saw myself as a weak and useless person, I countered by saying that I had many qualities and had studied hard, obtained diplomas and lived abroad. I felt he was trying to demolish my character, to dismantle me but I was still very fragile. I burst into tears and left.

"This is not achieving any purpose", I said in parting and he did not try to stop me. It was another dead end. Where was I to go from here?

*****

COMMENTARY 2

After my second episode of psychosis, I realised my experience in Paris was not a temporary aberration of the mind but an ongoing condition. I would have to face up to the reality of my illness. It was evident that the medical profession were not going to give me any support other than drug prescriptions. There was no dialogue between us. I would have to search by myself for a coping strategy.

My reading of the Swiss psychologist Carl Gustav Jung had taught me there was such a thing as the unconscious mind so I turned my mind in this direction. The voices during my first episode of schizophrenia in Paris had told me I was naive and needed educating. I decided therefore to study part time of an evening at Birkbeck College, University of London and the course I chose was French Literature. This was my choice for two reasons: one I enjoyed French: two French literature is heavily influenced by Roman Catholicism and I was aware that religion played a large part in my episodes of psychosis. I wanted to hone the critical part of my mind in order to understand what my mind was really saying to me when I was ill.

The French philosopher Descartes method of doubt particularly influenced me. I agreed with him that it was easy to take 'brass and glass' for 'gold and diamonds'. In other words, I did not want to accept anything as true unless there were good grounds for doing so.

The first thing I doubted was that God was speaking to me when I was ill. The voices came from inside me. Yet they seemed to be more knowledgeable than I. My only explanation is that unconsciously we pick up a lot of information that our mind files in the deep recesses of the brain and when I am ill, my mind erupts and all this information spews forth. My study reinforced what the voices had said, that my religious understanding had many flaws. There is a lot of mythology or spiritual truth that is not meant to be taken literally. The French philosopher Voltaire said in his book 'The Philosophical Dictionary' that faith is the suppression of reason and the implicit means by which the Church maintains temporal power and covers up its own immorality.

I needed a religion that appealed to my sense of reason as well as my imagination. Although much of my early religious education had been psychologically damaging, nevertheless religion was a force to combat malevolent forces. During my experience of illness, I had met God and the devil – both were equally petrifying.

I set about dismantling my religious mindset. At first, I looked to the occult and the East. I visited three psychics but was not impressed by their readings. The last psychic I visited told me that in a previous life I had been a victim of the holocaust and my American penfriend/boyfriend from New York State had been a German soldier. Our affair had been to resolve past grievances. This made me feel uneasy and I doubted her wisdom in telling me such a story.

I found Buddhism more helpful. The Buddha says we are what we think and I was conscious that there was a lot of psychic debris in my mind that needed cleansing. But the path to enlightenment was too complex for me to follow. I tried various forms of meditation and yoga to no avail.

I turned to Christianity again after reading a book by a Hindu who stated that it was a shame that in the West, we do not appreciate the wealth that lies within our own religion of Christianity.

From here I was led to a wonderful book 'The Golden String', by Bede Griffiths a Benedictine monk. He was a convert to Roman Catholicism, yet was aware of its violent past. As a young boy he had had a spiritual experience the memory of which had never left him. I could identify with his misgivings about the violent history of Christianity, for as a teenager, I had left the Roman Catholic Church on learning of the Inquisition. Also, I had known a timeless spiritual moment on a mountain top on my first trip to Switzerland. The beauty of that moment has never left me. 'The Golden String' was my Ariadne's thread that led back towards catholic spirituality and the eventual practice of contemplative prayer as a means of rest for my mind.

At University the medieval story of Yvain caught my interest. Here a knight who breaks his word, is humiliated falls into madness. – he is reduced to a primitive animal state but through his trials emerges a new and better man. I felt a parallel with my own situation. Schizophrenia had reduced me to the pits of my being. I had felt primeval forces at work on me as well as more sophisticated forces that open my hereto-closed mind to ideas I had not contemplated before. Like Yvain, I wanted to emerge a stronger better person.

The study of literature completely engaged my mind, and I felt less the sense of failure that was the by-product of schizophrenia. I did well in my studies. I felt empathy with the emotional turmoils of the fictional characters in the books I was reading. I saw in literature what I had met in psychosis. Literature was a world akin to my world of insanity. Moreover, in the philosophy of Voltaire there was a spirit of tolerance and true religion. However, when it came to the exams, the stress of wanting to succeed was triggering my symptoms and I had to abandon the course.

* * * * *

EPISODE 3

LONDON WINTER 1990/1991

The gangster raised the gun and fired. I felt the thud of the bullet against my skull. I had sat near the window in the lamplight of my bedroom so as to give him a clear view. It was a virtual reality killing. My fear and my courage not to run away had been real. I had paid the price for leaving my ex Italian husband. I must still have had guilt feelings for leaving him on bad terms. I felt electric shocks to my head. My circuits were blowing. But strangely the animosity I had harboured for a long time against my husband dissipated.

The next day Edith Piaf came and comforted me. We sang the song 'No, No Regrets'. I particularly liked singing 'Je m'en fous du passé' – Fuck the past. On a more solemn note we went and paid our respects to those Jews who lost their lives in the holocaust at the memorial at Gladstone Park. I also remembered those burned by the Roman Catholic Church by the Inquisition. We then continued on to Neasden to the pub that I had been told was the local IRA pub. I bought some matches at the Asian newsagents. There was a picture of the Acropolis on it. Greek fire – Greek fire was democracy. Edith and I smoked for peace and democracy in Northern Ireland outside the Irish pub.

I continued on to the library. There was a book on South Africa and the letters ANC came into my mind. This I translated to Ankh the Egyptian symbol for life.

Everything was taking on wider associations. Back at home television aggressively invaded my mind. The Gulf War had started. I was a nuclear bomb – the final deterrent. Only if I could keep my mind in balance would the war not cascade into a global conflict. A Buddhist monk came and showed me how to concentrate, and in my mind's eye I changed the number 4 on the television channel panel into a cross – the symbol of Christ's humanity – thus enabling me to maintain stability and preventing a nuclear holocaust.

* * * * *

It was winter and snow was falling. Mum and Dad packed me off to work, not grasping that I was ill. Work and routine gave the appearance of normality. The train was overcrowded and stuffy. We were packed like sardines and I was suffocating. I descended at Finchley Road instead of my usual station for the office. Pocahontas was waiting for me. We were to lead all the tribes, the Celts, the Bedouin, the Zulu and many more in a dance for peace and safety during these turbulent times. We sang as we danced round London and I smoked a cigarette for peace in the American Indian tradition at each religious site we passed. The tribes were a security belt for the world, and we allied telepathically during times of danger. We invoked the good spirits, the forces that could combat evil and war is evil.

I arrived at Hyde Park. It was deserted. I crossed the virgin snow leaving heavy footprints. The Sun was a ball of yellow in the sky. The shimmering ball transmuted into a human face. It was the face of Yul Brynner dressed in the uniform of a Chinese Communist. He spoke of the plight of the Chinese people. Unless the world dealt fairly with Communist China their land would be threatened by famine. Famine leads to war. My head was a human aerial which transmitted his words to an unknown respondent. The face faded. I smoked another cigarette to mark the end of the pow wow.

I made my way to the office in Lambeth and arrived mid-morning. My colleagues could see that I was unfit for work and sent me home. I walked from Lambeth to Victoria Station but in my mind's eye I was being carried by my dead Scottish Grandmother. A Protestant carrying a Roman Catholic. We passed by Westminster Abbey, the Methodist Hall and the Roman Catholic Cathedral – our union expressed a deep desire for Christian Unity.

I got lost in the maze of Victoria tube station but eventually found my way to Green Park and home – Neasden - labelled an immigrant area; but I saw it as a truly international township – there were Asians, West Indians, Irish, English and many more. I lived in the New Jerusalem – the world Christ died for – the global village that the world should become.

Soon after, as I could not keep up with the whizzing speed of my thoughts, I asked my doctor to send me to the hospital. Mum and Dad took me to Central Middlesex Hospital. As I was being examined by the doctor an anchor came flying through the window and embedded itself in my head. I found I could no longer count backwards. The whole mechanism of my mind was out of synchronisation.

In the hospital I felt as if I had been abandoned to hell but I did not want to stay with my family either because they start to panic when I have a turn. The world about me seemed in turmoil and the shock lightening pains in my head were too much to bear. I was terrified of electricity because in my confusion I associated the source of my pain with electric light. I wanted darkness and peace but come evening all around was bustle and burning artificial light.

After the confusion of the night I awoke next morning in the hospital to see the sun shining bright high up in the blue sky. Its invisible rays filtered through the window and lit the end of my bed. Slowly melting snow glistened on the rooftops. It was a treat for my eyes, especially after the harsh electric light of the night before. There was no more pain and confusion and my heart leaped with joy and renewed courage. I felt sensitive to a Divine presence in the world linking me to a unified whole or eternal design. I melted like the snow into the expanse of what, I suppose, one can only call God.

I sat cross-legged on my bed and drank in the beauty of it all – not only with my eyes but also deep in the depths of my being. I'd been elevated from one level of existence to another. I was filled with a joy in all creation – alone but at one with the world.

I don't know why I felt linked to something greater than myself. I wasn't feeling particularly religious that day – neither am I good. I always thought you had to pray for such moments but this came in answer to my need not a spoken prayer. This may well all be imaginative meandering, however I cannot deny the experience and can only trace it to a source beyond myself. In life we are always wanting in one way or another but in such moments all want is healed.

* * * * *

I fell into hospital routine. On the television news I learned that the IRA had exploded a bomb at Victoria Railway Station. I had been close to there only a few days before. I was glad to be safely away from the dangers of the city where I worked.

I was hyperactive and elated whilst in hospital. I understood how it was possible to face such terrors as death without fear for I felt united to a power beyond myself. I felt I was experiencing my common humanity with my fellow patients.

I made friends with a suicidal patient. In speaking to him, I took my lines from that great Hollywood film 'It's a Wonderful Life'.

"You love your grandchildren, don't you?"

"Yes" he replied.

"Just think if you had never been born, they would not exist. Your Life has meaning. Even though your wife and children reject you, remember you are the seed of your grandchildren."

This simple statement gave him something to hold onto and we became constant companions. There is often camaraderie between patients and if we are well enough we support each other.

There was quite a lot of freedom on the ward and I could come and go as I pleased. Once on my return to the ward an excited fellow patient wanted to speak to me urgently. He grabbed me and pulled me into an empty room. There he exposed himself to me. I surprised myself by not being shocked or afraid. He wanted me to fondle him. To his astonishment, I simply thanked him for his attentions and told him I was in love with somebody else and left. I did not report the incident, there is always the fear that the medical staff might assume it was symptomatic of my illness. My assailant did not bother me again. In normal circumstances I would have been terrified, but the elation I was experiencing made me pay no heed to danger.

The doctors had prescribed sulphiride as an alternative to the heavy-duty stelazine that I had been prescribed previously. Sulphiride was supposed to be a less dangerous drug. At first all was well, but after six months I had stopped menstruating which for a woman can give rise to problems in later life. After discussion, the doctors stopped all medication, which led to me eventually experiencing another relapse.

* * * * *

COMMENTARY 3

Psychotic insanity has taught me the human capacity to think in images. This inner world registers many experiences which would appear beyond the grasp of the rational mind. But this does not mean there is no relation at all to real life. But you need to find a key to interpret this fund of images. Saints see angels, Jesus or Mary. I met Edith Piaf, Pocahontas and Yul Brynner. Our unconscious will speak to us in a language we can understand. But my apparent yearning for a new world order and a morally perfect world is not far from that of the Christian message.

The imagination of the beholder always determines what is seen. The apparition could well be an extra-terrestrial which has become part of the folklore of our evolved culture. In the end it is the effect of the apparition on the viewer that matters. We clothe it in a form that is meaningful to ourselves but that does not mean the vision is infallible nor simply an illusion. It is the unconscious communicating in its language of myth and symbol. There is an objective reality to the emergence of chimera into our consciousness and it perhaps can be seen as a psychological mirror of our inner selves.

In the psyche are interwoven all the memories and responses to our life experiences. When I am ill, I awake to a deeper quality of existence despite the pain and exhaustion that it causes. It is a journey into the shadows and mystery of my own personality.

Beyond myself, I had felt an osmosis of feeling and thoughts between myself and the entities I had encountered and a fundamental connection between all living beings. For this reason, I pursued my interest in Christian spirituality and I went away to a Carmelite Priory to learn how to pray.

I was taught Centering Prayer which is a form of contemplative prayer. Contemplative prayer is silent prayer where the mind is freed of the excessive dependence of thinking. It leads to the release of unconscious emotional material and allows the cleansing of psychic debris which impedes our emotional equilibrium. Honest confrontation with the shadows of our psyche is less painful and destructive than avoidance. – a form of divine therapy. It also teaches us to have a right relationship with God but I will not go into the religious aspects here.

After my flirtation with Eastern religions and forms of meditation which had been to no avail, with centering prayer I experienced an immediate success. In the quiet of the cloister chapel, I experienced that timeless moment where eternity is now – the present moment. I found this healing and knew I had at last found the path for me. I have now practised centering prayer for over many years and as a coping strategy with my illness it helps slow down my over active mind and calms any paranoia. But at this juncture, I was simply a novice who by chance was given a hopeful start.

The discipline of centering prayer was to lead to change the habits of my mindset. After the rest of centering prayer, I experienced a freedom from my emotional turmoils. I felt less programmed by society and had a better perspective on life and myself. My judgement about what was good and harmful in my life developed. I knew my illness was not going to disappear but my courage to cope with it grew. Medication in schizophrenia has it part to play but it is only one aspect of the remedy. Our attitude towards the illness is crucial to managing the condition.

$$* * * * *$$

EPISODE 4

LONDON AUTUMN 1992

I had just come back from the Church social club with a friend. We had not really enjoyed the evening. I had not drunk port and lemon for a long time and it had upset my stomach; but I was feeling better now. My friend Rosetta stayed for coffee then went. All the family were in bed. I was too hyperactive for sleep and felt strangely elated. My brain was glowing inside my head. With my mind I could reach out beyond our three-dimensional world into a further dimension. An Irish man appeared – a rover who I took to be a distant relative of mine. My grandfather's unknown father perhaps? He did not appear in corporal form but as a beautiful circle of light that you could describe as a halo. He had come to give me reassurance and a message.

"There is Gaud".

I wrote the message down as if I had the gift of automatic writing. It was my hand but not my mind dictating the words. There was a two-fold meaning to the message.

'Gaud' comes from the Old French and Latin meaning joy and delight. So, one meaning was there is joy – joy is God and God is an experience. A form of consciousness.

Secondly 'Gaud' in modern day English means cheap trinket or bauble. This meant I must be careful to separate the gold in my mind from the dross. Hold nothing true until there are established grounds for believing it true. This latter meaning was very good advice echoing Descartes.

Overnight I gradually descended from elation into hell. Hell was television. My parents put on videos to distract me. Cary Grant was a favourite of mine. The films were no longer in colour but in black and white and Cary Grant was the devil who was there to challenge me. I was the suffering Job of the bible and I was sorely tried. I felt if I could watch the film unto the end, I would rise from my pit but I went through immense fear and anxiety as part of the process. I took solace in the thought that from hell the only way was up.

Although I could sit through videos, I could not watch television programmes especially the news. I felt I was on trial by the television presenters. My every thought was analysed.

I wanted world peace; I wanted cosmopolitan Neasden to be the New Jerusalem. But I was just a flawed human as full of prejudices as the next person. This racked my conscience. I needed to break out from my social conditioning. Nonetheless I saw a vision – the mountains of Switzerland rose up and flew to the walled city of Jerusalem in Israel. That was the answer to the Middle East conflict – for Jerusalem to become a neutral international city of peace.

My agitated condition was worrying my parents but they were loath to let me go into hospital again. That would be admitting defeat. I knew hospitalisation was the only way forward. The four walls of the house could not accommodate all my mental energy, and my parents' anxiety caused them at times to be aggressive. How could they know that when I was staring at the ceiling, I was seeing an allegory of the evolution of the species. How could they know how frightening it had been for me to experience my body completely paralysed with just my brain functioning. And how I had seen an appalling crucifixion that had turned into a myriad of stars as if indicating the birth of the universe.

* * * * *

The hallucinations exhausted me and I wanted rest. I needed medical help and despite my parents' misgivings sought my GP'. She sent me to Central Middlesex hospital but there were no beds available at Central Middlesex, so the doctor there sent me to Ealing hospital with a letter of instruction for my medical care.

I expected as after the previous two times to get immediate relief. I was in for a shock. Contrary to what my doctor at Central Middlesex had prescribed I was put on haloperidol which made me constantly restless and in need of perpetual motion. At first, I felt I had experienced a heavy hazy feeling of being drugged which made me feel quite ill, then came anxiety and the need for continual movement. Only contemplative prayer which helped still my mind and slow dance classes gave any respite. My suffering was as acute as my illness had been. When I complained of the bad side effects, I was told I would get used to it. But they were wrong. I never did get used to it. Several other patients were complaining about their medication. It was assumed that they were just being difficult.

The nurses informed my mother that I was not making any progress and that I was anti-social. I did not conform to their narrow model of 'normality'. They did not seem to understand that I was in distress and that it was from the haloperidol not my condition. Mum told me I would have to play by their rules to get released. By playing a few games of scrabble with the nurses in the day room I was rewarded with the prize of a weekend at home.

At home the restlessness was still unrelenting but I was grateful for the haven of my own room. I knew I needed to leave the hospital and speak to my doctor at Central Middlesex. I had not had such a difficult time since the bad effects of the heavy mediation in Paris. It was the medication and not me at fault but I also knew no one at Ealing hospital would listen.

When I return to Ealing hospital, I conformed to what the medical establishment considered normal behaviour despite my suffering. It was an act of sheer will on my part. The nurses told my mother I had greatly improved but I was only after my ticket out of the hospital.

At my outpatients' appointment back at Central Middlesex hospital, I told the doctor of the bad side-effects I was experiencing on the medication. He told me I should not have been put on haloperidol as he had instructed stelazine and procycladine for the side effects. He changed my prescription and within six weeks I had my life back.

* * * * *

COMMENTARY 4

The brain is a bio-computer and consciousness is essentially chemical in nature. I have always found it ironic the people spend enormous sums of money on illegal drugs to send themselves on trips and I have had to spend money on medication so as not to go off on a trip.

The brain is stored in the hardware of the human skull whereas the software – consciousness – is anywhere and everywhere. We are creatures of both mind and spirit. Human consciousness, like the universe, is expanding and as yet we do not know where the limits might lie. Consciousness is still largely unchartered territory. It is an inner and outer cosmos marked by our own experience.

Although it is now well established medically that there is a biological cause for schizophrenia, this does not mean we should not investigate the psychological meaning and significance of schizophrenic hallucinations. I maintain that hallucinations, like dreams, can be interpreted with reason.

Dreaming is normal so why do we label hallucinations as 'mad'.

Hallucinations have all the qualities of waking reality and are perhaps a means by which the psyche attempts to reprogramme our lives in order to find stability in a world in which we who live with schizophrenia are poorly adapted. I am conscious that I am two persons – my professional persona and my true self. In this life we are all subject to social conventions with which we may or may not agree. Society's models for living can be small and inhibiting. Most of our everyday experience is programmed and mechanical and often prevents us from becoming our authentic self. Hallucinations map out another reality, which is perhaps an esoteric process to make us change our life pattern.

A disability is not something with which people are very familiar. There is a huge lack of understanding about mental illness especially as there are no outward physical signs. People therefore tend not to take our problems seriously. We are often told to pull ourselves together and blamed for bringing the illness on ourselves. The stigma schizophrenia is a barrier to rehabilitation and our feelings are dismissed.

People who live with schizophrenia need time to re-adjust to society after a psychotic episode. They need to progress at their own pace. Pushing someone with schizophrenia to take up his or her former life too early may be counterproductive and hinder recovery. Going back to work, particularly to a stressful job could well lead to anxiety and the risk of relapse. As someone who lives with schizophrenia, I personally need time by myself and plenty of sleep. I try to balance this with some social activity.

The advent of schizophrenia which struck unexpectedly, made me change my lifestyle. The searing nature of my illness was a clear indication that I had to change direction if I was to find health. The process of auto analysis and reappraisal of my life, which had its terrible moments, became my means of recovery. It was this progression not prescriptions that made the experience easier to bear and less threatening.

* * * * *

EPISODE 5

LONDON AUTUMN 1994

Dad had died. My good friend John had died. Both from heart attacks. I had lost the two men who in the world loved me the most.

I was under stress at work. I worked for a boss and had as well two line managers above me. My boss was a controversial personality and this brought me into conflict with my line managers. I could not keep them all happy. I broke down.

The hallucinations were at first auditory. They spoke to me from the other side of the computer. My colleagues at work could see I was confused so I was asked to take some time off work and rest. I saw my doctor she gave me a sick certificate.

I enjoyed the freedom of being off work but could not stay in the confines of the house. At times I had the illusion that it was an incinerator that would burn me up if I did not escape.

One afternoon I took off and headed from Neasden to Westminster Abbey on foot. Places of religious significance were often my goal at such times. I ran like a comet across London.

On my journey, many spiritual entities tried to take me off my route. They were testing me. The traffic whirled by me at great speed and crossing the road was dangerous. Although I had no map, I trusted that somebody would watch over me and guide me to my destination of the Abbey.

When I reached the Abbey, I expected something momentous to happen. It didn't. This was a disappointing anti-climax so I went home.

Back in my room my mind kept churning in turmoil. Neasden was the New Jerusalem. I was in telepathic contact with all the tribes who still had the gift of the old ways. I was a link in a chain of communication with Zulus, Bedouin, the American Indians and Gypsies. We were a safety belt for the world. At the first sign of danger we awoke to our innate abilities to warn each other that our world was in danger.

Together we could transform the hostile negative forces that were threatening the world. I felt akin to all humanity.

In my reveries, I slept in the cool dark depths of the earth. The soil was black and fertile. I felt the presence of a monk who protected me. I felt safe.

Music was a stimulus. I danced out with the stars and felt tremendous energy flowing through my body. I became pure light – no mere edifice of flesh and bone but shot through with a vibrancy of life. I experienced the freedom of flying through the cosmos with a soul mate, and the harmony of being part of a beautiful patterned universe where I had my place. There was order in the chaos. I was a participant in the evolving universe – fully awakened and responsive to life.

The psychosis ran its course and eventually I returned to normality. My medication had not prevented a relapse but this time I had not felt the need to admit myself to hospital. I had undergone a process of inward disintegration which had led to eventual reintegration. I had come through and my mind had been opened to an existence so near yet so infinitely far away. ******

COMMENTARY 5

Schizophrenia is a disease of the brain but it is also a reaction to circumstances. I had suffered bereavement. I was under stress at work. But my failing brain had also opened my mind to a new consciousness that was healing. My flight into the eternal gave me hope of an afterlife where dad and John now resided. I believe death is an altered stated of consciousness. I believe schizophrenia is an altered state of consciousness. The basic state may be cerebral dysfunction but it is also an inward journey that goes beyond the realm of the brain to an expanded consciousness. This time by experiencing a full psychotic journey without hospital intervention, I felt I had made a hopeful victory. Perhaps the only true way out of psychosis is to struggle through it.

Religion is deeply psychological and a recurring theme in my psychotic experiences. It expresses our oneness with the cosmic whole (God). In our society of the nuclear family and where emphasis is on the individual, we often feel alienated and cut off from our common humanity with others. Religion should be a reassuring experience. Too often it is a damaging discipline where we live in fear of God, the ultimate policeman.

Some people believe the basis for God's existence is to answer prayers. Any pain or suffering they experience is an indication that something is wrong with God or them. We want to live in an Eden but we live in a fallen world. Eden was a state of childlike innocence. I'm personally glad that Eve gave Adam the apple. It is not Eve's fault that 'freewill' has been translated into 'licence to kill'.

Life does not always follow our scripts. Suffering happens but not always necessarily for a reason or because God is displeased with us – it is simply bad luck. Bad luck cannot be explained. A more mature relationship with divinity is to understand that God's hands and feet in this world, are we human beings. It is the collective responsibility of society to work to alleviate suffering. That is the challenge. Suffering and sacrifice are an inevitable part of life and can be transformative but not as a constant mode of life. I had to strike out by myself to find coping strategies for my condition, though I was fortunate enough to have family support for my material needs. However appropriate social support systems should be in place to lighten the load if self-help is to work well. Far too many mentally ill patients are bereft of any such structure and cannot be expected to take responsibility for their own lives and future until appropriate help is available.

Psychology is the new cult of our age to respond to the illness of the human condition. Therapy is an unloading process for emotional healing. Schizophrenia is a dramatic unloading of the unconscious and if we ignore the issues that come to light, they will only reassert themselves until we do take notice. Although I cannot change the world, as is my wish when I am ill, I can change myself.

We can be safe and at home with our own psyches. We just need to understand the language of the unconscious so we can experience liberation instead of fear and enslavement. It is denial and repression that causes destructive symptoms.

* * * * *

EPISODE 6

HERTFORDSHIRE - SUMMER 2000

Mum had been killed in an accident and soon after my brother Colin died of a heart attack. I eventually became ill.

I awoke suddenly to a latent form of consciousness that rendered me telepathic. I conversed with inner voices who took the guise of people from the media, politics and colleagues from work.

Again, arose the fantasy that I was a telepathic link in a chain and together via thought transference we could influence for the better, people and world events. There were others who worked against this. I was neutral and non-aligned. Above patriotism and political and religious affiliations. I wanted a better world for all.

I believed it was important that I was not found so as to carry on this secret work. I marked out a safe ground by walking around the village - my New Jerusalem. The most important landmark was the library. In the past it had been a church. This signified that I was to change course for a while from my religious research to more secular matters. However, I found my practice of contemplative prayer, which had the effect of calming my mind, a great aid during my indisposition. The bombardment of thoughts, the invasion of my mind by television or hostile emanations could be exhausting. However, I could cope with videos which were vehicles to explain my personal, religious and political beliefs that I felt were on trial. What I was seeing and the actual action on the screen were two very different scripts.

The telepathic network is a kind of great game. I encountered all manner of people: the Masons, the Mafia. Friendlier entities were a Lama who lives on the other side of the Universe and a Zen Buddhist who appeared in the guise of Yul Brynner. I also felt contact with my departed parents and brother.

I believed my thoughts were transparent to the people in the village so I tried to mask my thoughts by thinking in French and German. However, after a few days they got interpreters in. I also turned to music and song to stop the invasion of the privacy of my mind. Thinking in a foreign language and song slowed down my thought processes and I was better able to cope with the delirium.

During the psychosis, my senses of sight and hearing became more acute. The sound of a car or the babble of voices was intolerable. My mind was working on two levels: reality in order to deal with the people I met in the real world and chimera. However, I could appear to be rather slow.

Matters of a personal nature were sorted out with spiritual beings – guardian angels without the wings. They are probably some kind of inner voice coming from my unconscious mind. I must admit they were quite insightful and helpful.

The spiritual beings helped me sort out my finances so I could see that working part-time could be economically viable. I felt that work had taken over my life and I wanted to break out of the monotonous routine.

They also told me to go and see my GP. I did not feel the doctor would take me seriously but they insisted so I went. She gave me a certificate for sick leave from work. In the end,

I was getting no better and on experiencing a panic attack, I phoned in desperation for an ambulance. I was taken to Hemel Hospital where I managed to calm down and they sent me home. As a result of this and action from my welfare officer at work, my GP referred me to Watford hospital for treatment.

At times I was like a silly small child who was always laughing and my head swayed to and fro like a horse. I saw myself as a humanised unicorn. The beauty of being a child is that it is a pure state of being not thinking. I had a twin unicorn and our minds were able to interlock and I felt complete.

There was also a dark side to the psychosis. I underwent moments when I felt I was under attack by hostile psychic forces. An oppressive weight the bulk of an anvil was on my head and I felt it could drive me insane. This I believed was a way for hostile forces to intimidate me.

I felt my stomach was a bulging sack of potatoes. This again was a deception by hostile psychic forces. Although I felt sated and slightly sick, I forced myself to eat. This dispelled the hallucination.

Witches were able to scramble my brain and cause me searing mental pain by stabbing me in the head with invisible daggers.

In the kitchen it was possible to experience my mind as a spring that was being over wound. I could only unwind by retracing my steps. It was rather like dancing the waltz backwards.

On a lighter note, two of my spiritual beings were able to stimulate me sexually by emanating energy in the form of light. This energy entered my body and gave me great pleasure. The French call climax la petite morte literally the little death. The ecstasy was so great that I indeed thought I could die. Things were scaled down to one spiritual being. This I could cope with. The brain is definitely the most important sexual organ in the human body. It may appear to the reader that this is an erotic fantasy and a symptom of sublimated sexuality. I personally feel at home with my sexuality and I know a healthy attitude towards sex is necessary for our psychological well-being. I found the experience liberating and this at least was safe sex.

* * * * *

During the latter part of my psychosis, I was an outpatient at Watford Hospital. The doctor changed my medication to one of the newer anti-psychotic drugs called olanzapine. The hallucinations gradually receded and I returned to normality.

* * * * *

COMMENTARY 6

A lot of my experiences during a psychotic crack up are personal and subjective but some are rooted in observable reality. There is some rhyme and reason to my behaviour when I am ill.

During my psychotic fantasies, I am a hero on a journey confronting the dragons of war and greed in our world. But mine is the heroism more of a martyr than a dragon slayer. Through my links with spiritual entities, I experience a sense of community that is perhaps lacking in my personal life. A community which I believe is evolving and whose path is world peace. I evolve by having my spiritual beings via all sorts of media - television, radio, telepathy, - challenge my prejudices. I work for world peace but declare war on myself. There is no shying away from the quest. My brain or is it my conscience will not let me rest. There is nowhere I can hide.

The voices or spiritual beings, wherever they come from have at times been insightful and galvanised me into making changes in my way of life. Schizophrenia has been beneficial to the point that it has brought about a realignment of my personality and spurred me on to find a new and better path. It has opened my mind to new ideas and I have grown into a fuller person. It has been a path from terror to enlightenment.

However, schizophrenia is not without it powerful dark side when all can seem lost especially if one is experiencing searing physical and mental pain. This is where appropriate understanding and medical care is needed. The newer anti-psychotic drugs are of important value in this respect and I do not relegate them to an inferior place. But I also feel my own coping strategies of contemplation and research and analysis of my psychoses have given me a greater self awareness and by acknowledging the chaos within, I am better equipped to cope with my symptoms when I am ill.

Mental agony is terrible because it cannot be communicated to anyone except the person who has suffered the same fate. People who suffer mental illness often feel diminished and of no value in the world's eyes. When illness strikes, people will often recede from their pain and suffering. Thereby they are driven inwardly into themselves and become prisoners of their own mind. The rejection and isolation can be overwhelming. At this point you can either quit the struggle or continue to wrestle with the mental anguish. It is possible to prevail against the unremitting suffering and dark despair.

*****

I have written down here an account of my psychotic fantasies which I have experienced during illness. In this way I no longer feel the prey of my illness. It has been an honest confrontation with my unconscious and by learning about breakdown, I have made a breakthrough. I still suffer from mental instability but now I can make sense of the experience. Confrontation with my inner world has brought me a greater familiarity with myself.

To quote the famous psychologist Carl Gustav Jung:

"I had to try and understand what had happened and to what extent my own experience coincided with that of mankind in general. Therefore, my first obligation was to probe the depths of my own psyche"

Memories, Dreams and Reflections.

In my life, I had experienced personal disillusionment. There was an early disappointment with religion when I found out about the crimes of the Inquisition. I could no longer trust the institution of the Church. I found out that governments are not always good and that the world was not a humane and free place to be. Humankind is still more skilled in the arts of war than the arts of peace. My relationships with my husband and lovers were a failure. The trauma of schizophrenia put an end to my international career. Early medical care did not come to my rescue. Real life was not how I wished it to be. For I long time I felt a powerless victim of my illness and an outsider in society. It was a painful stage.

A key move from despair to hope was my pursuit of knowledge. After my discovery of the unconscious through reading the autobiography of the Swiss psychologist Carl Gustav Jung, I studied literature part time at University and I learned all I could about mental illness. Study taught me that I was not simply 'mad'. What had happened was not my fault but the result of an illness. My experiences were not unique and I was not alone. In this way I rebuilt myself and my pain gave way to inquiry. I began to find schizophrenia an interesting subject that is much misunderstood.

I felt if I was attentive to the feedback from my psychotic fantasies, I could access the root of my illness and strengthen my ability to manage the condition. Once I had sifted through all the confusion, I could discern what my unconscious was telling me. My deep emotional feelings were silhouetted in my fantasies. By reflection I could put things into perspective.

My first duty was towards my own well-being. I had to accept my illness despite my melancholia at the damage it had done to me and from there negotiate a new approach to life. I took up study and writing as a means of self-expression. Over years the pain gradually receded. With the help of contemplative prayer, I have tried to integrate the warring components of my psyche so I can have the freedom to become my authentic self and thereby bring myself to wholeness and health. My method has been to open myself to the intuitive insights of my unconscious and try to relate to them by use of my reason. It is important that the reality of the experience is not accepted uncritically.

In this way, I no longer have a bleak view of myself as I did after my first two psychoses in 1984 and 1985 the first of which I tried to blank. Once you are free from the pressure of what other and society thinks you can be more relaxed with yourself. I try to dispel some to the stigma surrounding schizophrenia by being open about it.

* * * * *

A FINAL WORD

According to legend, because of Pandora's action in opening the forbidden box, evil was made manifest in the world. But hope quickly followed in its footsteps to aid a struggling humanity. Although there is as yet no cure for schizophrenia, there is hope for those who have to live with and manage the condition.

Often, we fear what we do not know and do not want to know what we fear. I have come to know myself through my experience of schizophrenia and I hope my book is a way of opening the Pandora's box on mental illness and letting a ray of hope shine for us all.

Mental illness does not discriminate it strikes across the divides of race, age, class and sexuality. Neither should society discriminate against those who live with mental illness. Mental illness is more about human experience than a medical category.

* * * * *

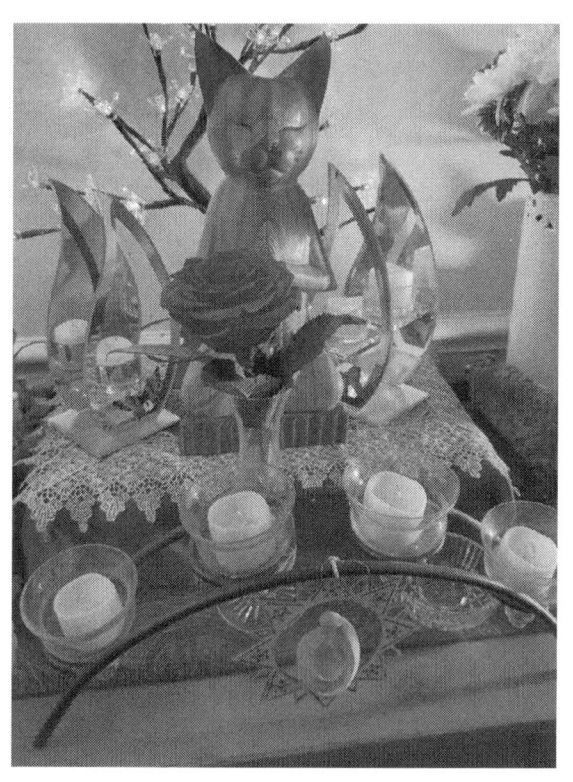